CONTE

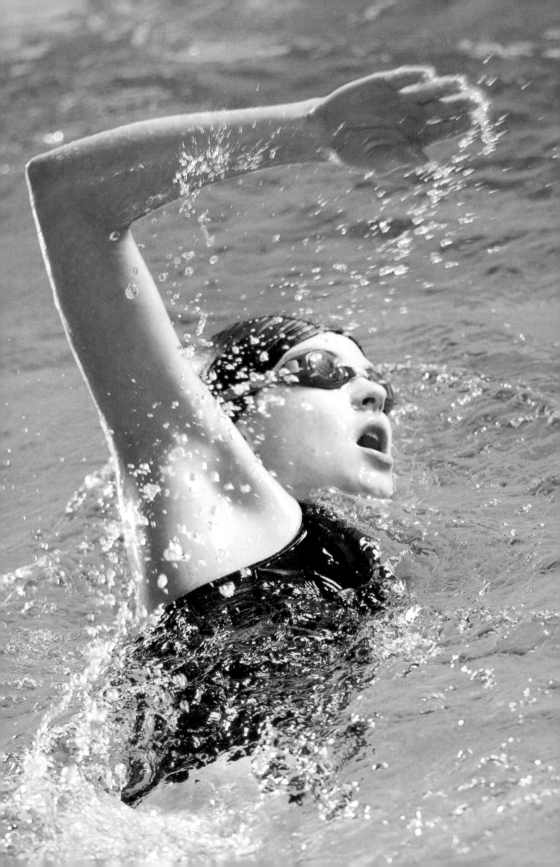

BENEFITS OF FITNESS SWIMMING

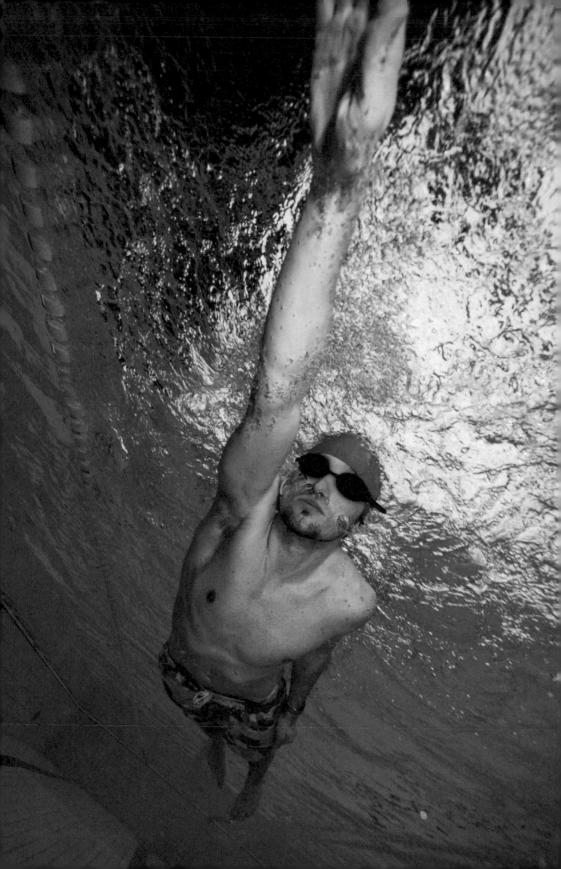

W hether you are a beginner working to increase your fun and fitness, or a veteran swimmer looking to add motivation and challenge into your training, the 100 organized swim sessions in *The Swimmer's Workout Handbook* are for you.

I've spent years doing organized swim workouts, or standing on the pool deck coaching a masters swim group, while at the same time noticing many of the other lap swimmers in the pool going back and forth, with no apparent plan. Consistent swimming of any sort will build—and then stabilize—your fitness, and is a fabulous non-weight-bearing activity. In order to get stronger and faster, without the mind-numbing boredom of staring at that black line, a well-planned, diverse workout is in order. *The Swimmer's Workout Handbook* gives you the new edge you are looking for, while putting big doses of variety into each workout.

Swimming improves core, muscular, and cardiovascular strength and endurance, all in a low-impact, gravity-free workout. If done two to several times per week, or as an addition to a multi-sport training regime, swimming helps maintain a healthy weight, heart, and lungs. These benefits are best realized within the diversity of your workouts. To increase your swim fitness it is optimal to vary intensity, interval distances, recovery, and strokes, all within one workout session. The diversity within a workout is what triggers the body to grow stronger, faster, and more proficient. Whether you only have time to swim 1000 meters/yards, or are up for 5000 at each session, *The Swimmer's Workout Handbook* organizes speed, distance, and technique into these 100 fun and challenging training sessions—putting vitality back into your pool time.

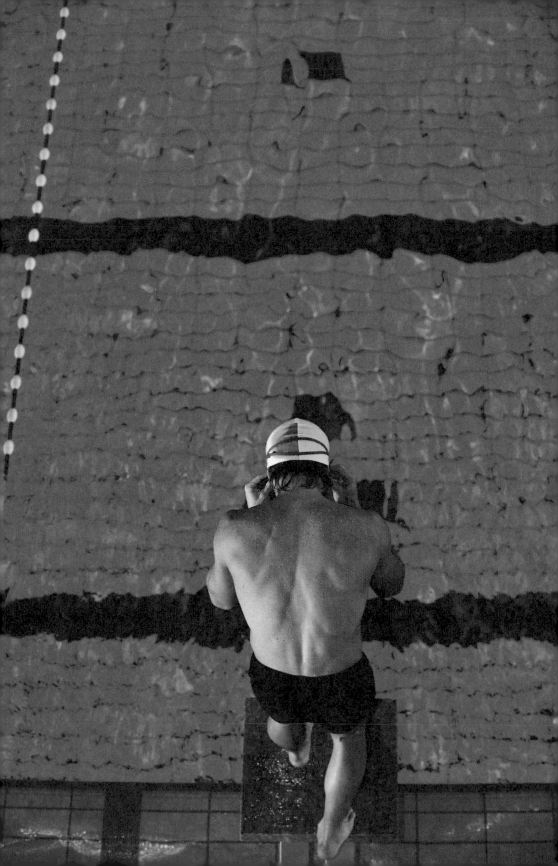

GENERAL TERMS AND GUIDANCE

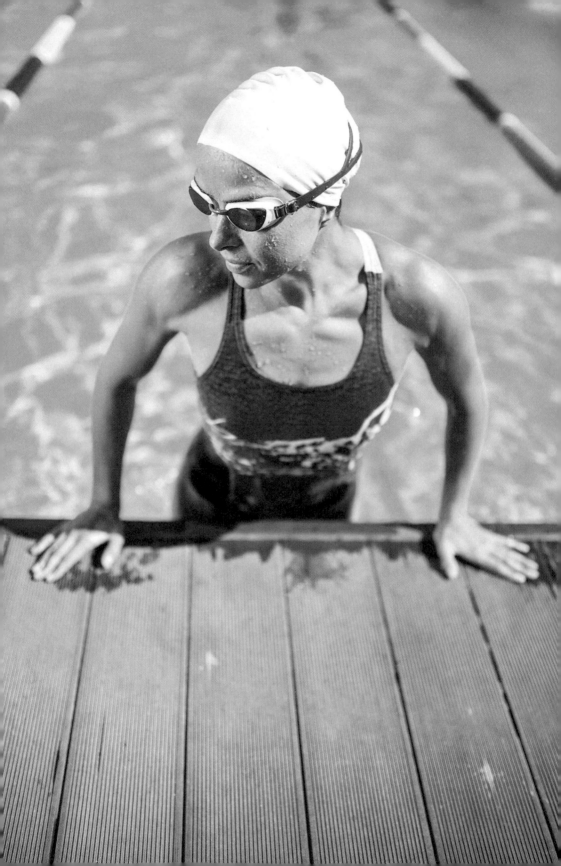

Gear Requirements

Swimsuit: There are too many types and brands of suits to list here, but the main objective is to find a suit that is comfortable, streamlined in the water, and that you enjoy wearing. Some use their suits to make a fashion statement at every workout, while others wear an inexpensive suit even after it starts to sag in the butt due to dissolving elastic. Whichever your style, choose a suit that feels comfortable in the water.

Goggles: Goggles not only protect your eyes in salt water or chemical-infused water, but they help you see clearly both above and below the water while swimming. Goggles need to fit your face and be comfortable to wear for long periods of time. If they are adjustable in the nose piece and head strap, you have a better chance of working them to prevent leaking or fogging. Try them on in the store. If they hug your eye area with ease, make the purchase. You may need to try a few pairs before you find the one brand that works on your face.

When testing the goggles in the water, adjust them to feel snug, but comfortable. Some goggles have fog-resistant residue built into each lens. Additional ways to prevent fogging are to spit in the lenses and swish the spit around, or use a defog product (as directed on the package), then dip them in water before putting them on. Try wearing the goggles for half or more of your swim workout without taking them off; they should feel comfortable after this length of time. If they start to bother your face or feel like they are causing discomfort on your eyes, adjust the strap to ease the pressure. If you can't relieve this discomfort or eliminate leaking or fogging, get another pair and start over.

For outdoor swimmers with eyes that are very sensitive to sunlight, opt for a darker lens. You can wear a lighter lens for early morning or evening swims, but you'll want the darker lens for midday swimming when there is a strong possibility that the sun will hit you in the face.

Swim cap: Your swim cap helps keep your head streamlined and insulated in the water and also keeps your hair out of your face. When you purchase a swim cap, choose one that doesn't pull your hair when you put it on, and stays on your head when swimming long distances. A popular choice is silicone. They are comfortable, longer lasting, and warmer than light-weight rubber swim caps, but they do cost a bit more. Some opt for lycra swim caps for comfort, but take note that water can move through a lycra cap, making your head much less streamlined in the water than a sealed rubber cap.

Earplugs: Some would consider earplugs to be optional, but for a few reasons, all swimmers should wear them. When your ear is regularly exposed to excess moisture, water can remain trapped in your ear canal. The skin inside can become waterlogged, diluting the acidity that normally prevents infection. The soggy skin will also more readily allow bacteria to penetrate your skin. Bacteria and fungi from contaminated water can grow and cause swimmer's ear, which is an infection of your outer ear and ear canal. All of the above can be prevented by using earplugs during your swimming workouts.

Earplugs are available in two varieties: soft moldable silicone plugs and pre-molded rubber plugs. As with goggles, earplug brand and type is a personal preference. Use the type that is comfortable for you and keeps the water out of your ears.

Kickboard: Use a kickboard for kick sets in training, but also learn to do kick sets without a board. When using a kickboard, wrap the fingers of both hands around the top of the board and extend your arms out and over your head. Your forearms will naturally rest on top of the board.

Pull buoy: Place the pull buoy between your legs at the top of your thighs. Using a pull buoy draws the legs up behind you and will help you focus on how your upper body affects your stoke.

Paddles: Paddles are most often used with a pull buoy, but you can play with using them without a buoy, as desired. There are a variety of paddle sizes and styles to choose from. If you are new to paddles, choose a smaller paddle to start. Using swim paddles not only requires you to move your arms and hands effectively through the water, but they will help you gain strength. However, only use swim paddles if you have no shoulder issues as they can put extra stress on the shoulder.

Fins: Use fins or short fins to strengthen your legs and teach yourself proper body position in the water (particularly when doing drills). Just like paddles or the pull buoy, fins can be an excellent teaching aid but should not be the focus of your swim workouts. If you are looking to generate a more productive kick, focus on proper drill technique, or increase your heart rate a bit, try using the short or chopped-off style of fins for a swim or drill set within each workout.

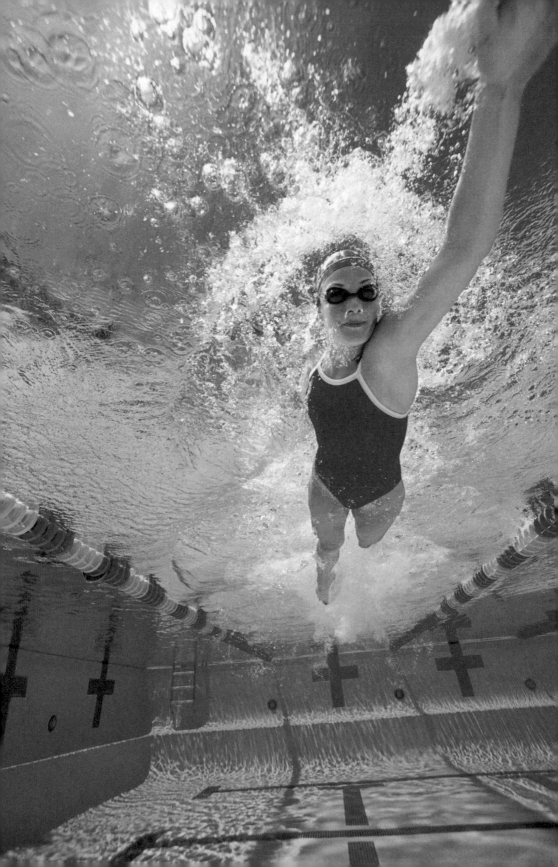

Helpful Workout Terminology

1-4, 5-8: This refers to the first through fourth, and the fifth through eighth intervals in a set.

6-3-6 drill: 6 beat kick on your left side with left arm extended, 3 strokes, 6 beat kick on your right side with right arm extended. Repeat.

Aerobic: In the presence of oxygen.

Anaerobic: Without oxygen. Anaerobic exercise uses muscles at a high intensity and a high rate of work, for a short period of time. Anaerobic exercise helps us increase our muscle strength and sustain higher speeds for longer periods of time.

Anaerobic threshold: Onset of blood lactate accumulation during exercise, or the exercise intensity at which lactic acid is produced faster than it can be metabolized. Also referred to as "lactate threshold".

Build: Progressively increase the speed of the interval.

Build each: Progressively increase the speed of each interval within a set.

Butterfly: Stroke swam on your front with both arms moving simultaneously, accompanied by two dolphin kicks for every stroke cycle.

Backstroke: Upside down freestyle stroke with a flutter kick.

Breaststroke: Stroke swam on your front with arms moving simultaneously to the front and underneath the swimmer with no torso rotation and accompanied by a whip or frog kick (see breast kick).

Breathe every: During freestyle, take a breath every designated stroke (for example, every 3rd, 5th, or 7th stroke).

Broken at: Pause the interval at the designated distance (such as 25, 50, 100, etc.) for the assigned rest interval, such as :05R (see "Time" on page 14).

Catch up drill: Recovery arm 'catches up' with the extended arm at the top of the stroke before the extended arm pulls through.

Choice of stroke: Your choice of whichever stroke you wish.

Descend the set: Progressively increase the speed of each interval in a set.

Evens: 2nd, 4th, 6th, etc., intervals within a set.

Fastest average: The fastest pace you can average for the given set and rest interval.

Fastest time: Your fastest time for the designated interval.

Finger tip drag drill: Freestyle with an exaggerated high bent-elbow recovery and relaxed lower arm, causing your finger tips to drag along the top of the water.

Fist drill: Freestyle with each hand in a fist.

Freestyle or front crawl: Swim on your front with each arm alternating, above the water, above your head, to the front, then underneath your body and accompanied by a flutter kick. Generally regarded as the fastest stroke.

Head up drill or water polo stroke: Freestyle with the head slightly above the water line, with eyes forward.

Heart rate: The number of times a heart beats in a minute. See also maximum heart rate and recovering heart rate.

High-end aerobic: The upper end of an athlete's aerobic training level.

Individual medley (IM): An interval or event with the following order of strokes: butterfly, backstroke, breaststroke, freestyle.

Interval: Repetition of a prescribed workload followed by periods of recovery or low activity. For example, in the set 4x50, each 50 is an interval within the set.

Kick: If just the word 'kick' is used, do flutter kick unless otherwise designated, or:

> **Dolphin kick:** Used when doing butterfly. Legs and feet move side-by-side in an undulating manner, up and down.

> **Breast kick:** Used when doing breaststroke. Keeping your knees about body width apart, bring your heels up towards your butt while flexing your feet, then whip your feet and lower legs to each side then back together while facing the soles of your feet together as much as possible.

> **Back kick:** Used when doing backstroke. Flutter kick on your back.

Flutter kick: Used when doing freestyle. The kick starts from the hips, then in an up and down undulating motion, propulsion transfers through each leg, then ankle, and pointed foot as they alternate in pressing down toward the bottom of the pool.

Left arm drill: Swimming freestyle with just your left arm while the other arm is either extended overhead or at your side.

Locomotion: For a 300: 25 sprint/25 easy/50 sprint/50 easy/75 sprint/ 75 easy. For a 500: 25 sprint/25 easy/50 sprint/50 easy/75 sprint/75 easy/ 100 sprint/100 easy.

No board: Kick as designated, without a kick board, and with arms extended overhead.

Odds: 1st, 3rd, 5th, etc., intervals within a set.

Pacing: Executing a particular speed for a given distance and event.

Pull: Freestyle with a pull buoy between your thighs (no kick) and paddles (optional).

Right arm drill: Swimming freestyle with just your right arm while the other arm is either extended overhead or at your side.

Set: One group of repetitions of an exercise. For example: 4x50. This type of number grouping designates a set. In this example, you'll swim 50, 4 times as designated while taking the assigned amount of rest between each 50. A set can also be a grouping of short sets within a larger collection.

Stroke count: Count how many strokes you take per 25. An objective is to decrease this number over time.

Time: For example, ":10R" means 10 seconds of rest and "1:00R" means 1 minute of rest. If there is no rest interval designation, take as much rest as needed, while still challenging yourself.

Training level designation: Do the designated interval(s) at this level (for example, L2). See the Training Levels Chart on page 16 for more details.

Training Levels

Each training level in the Training Levels Chart on page 16 is described by:

- What it is used for

- One's "perceived exertion", using the Borg Perceived Exertion chart on page 18

- Corresponding heart rate (HR) range (see below)

Heart rate (HR) range is shown as an assigned "% of max" number. This number designates an HR range relative to your maximum HR. For example, 80% of max is 80% of your maximum HR. You can choose which method of evaluating your intensity level suits you; however, in order to use the "% of max" numbers within each level, you must know your max HR.

If you are not currently using a heart rate monitor or you have not tested for your max HR, use the Training Levels Chart on page 16 to decipher your workout efforts via how a level is used or by your perceived exertion (using the Borg Perceived Exertion Scale on page 18). It is important for you to become familiar with these workout levels and how they feel for you.

If you have a heart rate monitor and you know your max HR (*only* by taking a max HR test, *not* by using a formula), you can use your monitor to establish training intensity on the Training Levels Chart. Otherwise, use the additional information on the chart to establish your workout levels.

TRAINING LEVELS CHART

(See the Borg Perceived Exertion scale on page 18)

Level 1: Recovery

- *Used for*: Recovery, warm-up, cool-down, and baseline endurance

- *Perceived Exertion (PE):* 9-10; you can talk easily, effort is extremely easy

- *HR Range:* 65-75% of max

Level 2: Aerobic

- *Used for*: Improving aerobic, or oxygen utilization capacity, warm-up, cool down, and longer training and races

- *Perceived Exertion (PE):* 11-13; conversations are comfortable, effort is moderate to easy

- *HR Range:* 75-80% of max

Level 3: High-End Aerobic to Low Anaerobic

- *Used for*: Improving lactate system, intervals, tempo training, and long- to moderate-distance training and races

- *Perceived Exertion (PE):* 14-15; short conversations are possible, effort is moderate to challenging

- *HR Range:* 80-85% of max

Level 4: Lactate or Anaerobic Threshold

- *Used for*: Improving ability to mobilize lactate for longer periods, intervals, and moderate- to short-distance training and races

- *Perceived Exertion (PE):* 16-18; difficult to speak, effort is challenging to difficult

- *HR Range:* 85-90% of max

Level 5: Sub-Maximum to Maximum Effort*

- *Used for*: Training fast twitch muscles to develop power, strength and speed, intervals and sprint training and events

- *Perceived Exertion (PE):* 19-20; breathing is labored, effort is very difficult

- *HR Range:* 90-100% of max

* **Maximum HR** is pre-set, or genetic, and can be determined optimally through a max heart rate test. Maximum HR will decline with age. We cannot train our max HR to become higher, but we can train to be better at taking a max HR test.

BORG PERCEIVED EXERTION (PE) SCALE

The Borg Perceived Exertion (PE) Scale gives you an idea of how hard your exercise feels. Use the below scale to aid your efforts to work within the corresponding training levels designated for each workout on your training program:

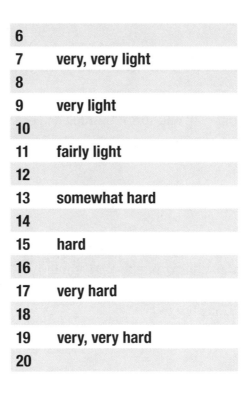

6	
7	very, very light
8	
9	very light
10	
11	fairly light
12	
13	somewhat hard
14	
15	hard
16	
17	very hard
18	
19	very, very hard
20	

SWIM WORKOUTS

NOTES: The distances of these swim workouts reference either meters or yards, whichever is relevant to the pool you use.

These workouts are for swimmers with a variety of athletic experience. The distance of the workouts you choose to execute will, in part, depend on how much time you have to devote to your swim time. Any workout distance, if practiced diligently, will give you increased skill and endurance. If you are looking to increase your swim fitness over time, we recommend starting with workouts in the 1000-2000 range and then increasing by increments of 200-300 meters/yards each week, as your schedule allows. If you have an option to work on your swim technique with a coach or swim instructor, we recommend you do so, as this will greatly enhance your competency in the water.

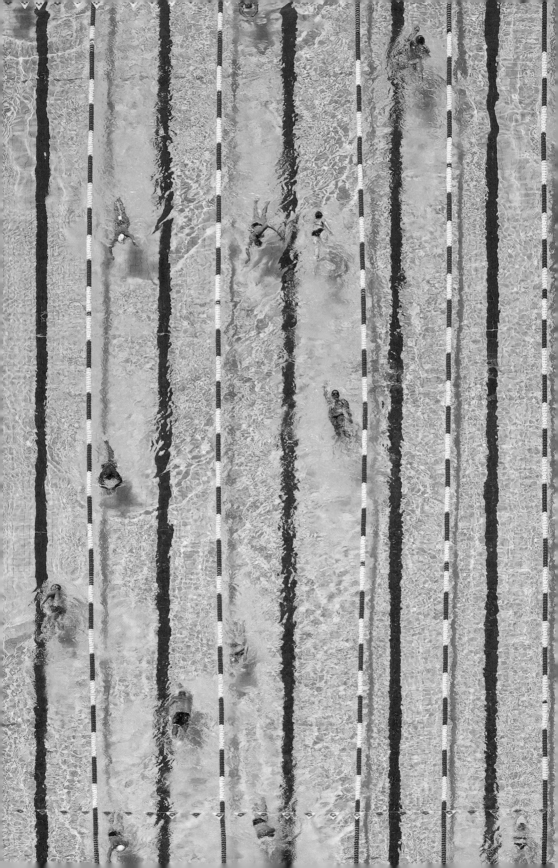

Swim Workouts: 1000-2000 Yards or Meters

NOTE: The distances of these swim workouts reference either meters or yards, whichever is relevant to the pool you use.

| 100 freestyle (L2) 100 kick (L2) | WARM-UP |

4x50; 25 catch up drill/25 freestyle
  w/:15R

200 alternate; 25 fingertip drag
  drill/25 freestyle

200 pull (L3)
100 freestyle (L4)

| 100 kick (L2) | COOL-DOWN |

TOTAL: 1000

L1: Recovery; **L2**: Aerobic; **L3**: High-End Aerobic to Low Anaerobic;
L4: Lactate or Anaerobic Threshold; **L5**: Sub-Maximum to Maximum Effort

2

200 choice of stroke (L2)
2x100 kick (L3) w/:10R

2x100 freestyle build each w/:15R
200 pull (L3)

100 catch up drill
100 choice of stroke (L2)

TOTAL: 1000

3

≈≈≈

200 choice of stroke (L2)
100 kick (L2)

2x50 6-3-6 drill w/:15R

2x200 freestyle w/:20R;
   1 (L3)
   2 (L4)
4x25 freestyle (L5) w/:15R

100 choice of stroke (L2)

TOTAL: 1000

L1: Recovery; L2: Aerobic; L3: High-End Aerobic to Low Anaerobic;
L4: Lactate or Anaerobic Threshold; L5: Sub-Maximum to Maximum Effort

4

≈≈≈

100 choice of stroke (L2)

2x100 kick (L3) w/:15R

**2x100; 50 finger tip drag drill/50
  catch up drill w/:15R**

200 freestyle (L4)

300 pull (L3)

200 choice of stroke (L2)

TOTAL: 1200

L1: Recovery; L2: Aerobic; L3: High-End Aerobic to Low Anaerobic;
L4: Lactate or Anaerobic Threshold; L5: Sub-Maximum to Maximum Effort

5
≋

200 choice of stroke (L2)

200 kick; 10 beat kicks on each side (L2)

2x100; 25 left arm drill/25 right arm drill/50 freestyle w/:15R

300 pull; breathe every 3rd stroke (L4)

8x25 freestyle (L5) w/:20R

100 choice of stroke (L2)

TOTAL: 1200

L1: Recovery; **L2**: Aerobic; **L3**: High-End Aerobic to Low Anaerobic;
L4: Lactate or Anaerobic Threshold; **L5**: Sub-Maximum to Maximum Effort

6
≋

200 choice of stroke (L2)
100 kick; 10 beats on each side (L2)

100 finger tip drag drill

50, 100, 200, 100, 50 freestyle (L4) w/:30R
8x25 w/:20R;
   1-4 freestyle (L5)
   5-8 IM order (L5)

100 freestyle (L2)

TOTAL: 1200

L1: Recovery; L2: Aerobic; L3: High-End Aerobic to Low Anaerobic;
L4: Lactate or Anaerobic Threshold; L5: Sub-Maximum to Maximum Effort

7

≋

200 choice of stroke (L2)
2x100 kick (L2) w/:10R

100 catch up drill

100 pull (L3)
100, 150, 100, 50 freestyle (L4) w/:20R
4x25 freestyle (L5) w/:20R

100 freestyle (L2)

TOTAL: 1200

L1: Recovery; **L2**: Aerobic; **L3**: High-End Aerobic to Low Anaerobic;
L4: Lactate or Anaerobic Threshold; **L5**: Sub-Maximum to Maximum Effort

8

200 choice of stroke (L2)
100 kick (L2)

100 fist drill

2x200 freestyle build each w/:30R
2x50 freestyle (L5) w/:30R
4x25 freestyle (L5) w/:10R
200 pull (L3)

200 choice of stroke (L2)

TOTAL: 1400

L1: Recovery; **L2**: Aerobic; **L3**: High-End Aerobic to Low Anaerobic;
L4: Lactate or Anaerobic Threshold; **L5**: Sub-Maximum to Maximum Effort

9

200 choice of stroke (L2)

4x50 kick; 25 back/25 choice of stroke (L3) w/:20R

3x200 freestyle descend the set w/:30R

300 pull locomotion

100 choice of stroke (L2)

TOTAL: 1400

L1: Recovery; L2: Aerobic; L3: High-End Aerobic to Low Anaerobic;
L4: Lactate or Anaerobic Threshold; L5: Sub-Maximum to Maximum Effort

10

200 choice of stroke (L2)

100 fist drill

2x100; 25 right arm drill/25 left arm
     drill/50 freestyle w/:10R

200 pull (L3)

4x50 kick (L5) w/:10R

4x75 freestyle (L4) w/:20R

2x50 freestyle (L5) w/:10R

100 choice of stroke (L2)

TOTAL: 1400

L1: Recovery; L2: Aerobic; L3: High-End Aerobic to Low Anaerobic;
L4: Lactate or Anaerobic Threshold; L5: Sub-Maximum to Maximum Effort

11

200 choice of stroke (L2)
2x100 kick (L2) w/:10R

3x100; 50 catch up drill/50 finger tip drag drill w/:10R

2x150 freestyle (L3) w/:10R
100 (L2), 4x25 (L5), 100 (L3) freestyle w/:15R

200 choice of stroke (L2)

TOTAL: 1500

L1: Recovery; **L2**: Aerobic; **L3**: High-End Aerobic to Low Anaerobic;
L4: Lactate or Anaerobic Threshold; **L5**: Sub-Maximum to Maximum Effort

12
≈≈≈

200 choice of stroke (L2)

100 catch up drill

200 pull (L3)

6x75 freestyle descend the set
w/:20R

150 freestyle; 50 (L3)/50 (L5)/50 (L3)
w/:20R

200; 50 backstroke/50
breaststroke/50 backstroke/50
breaststroke (L3)

200 choice of stroke (L2)

TOTAL: 1500

L1: Recovery; L2: Aerobic; L3: High-End Aerobic to Low Anaerobic;
L4: Lactate or Anaerobic Threshold; L5: Sub-Maximum to Maximum Effort

13
≋

200 choice of stroke (L2)
100 kick (L2)

100 6-3-6 drill

300 pull locomotion
3x100 freestyle (L5) w/:30R
300 kick (L3)
4x50 freestyle (L4) w/:20R

100 choice of stroke (L2)

TOTAL: 1600

L1: Recovery; L2: Aerobic; L3: High-End Aerobic to Low Anaerobic;
L4: Lactate or Anaerobic Threshold; L5: Sub-Maximum to Maximum Effort

14

300 choice of stroke (L2)

100 kick (L2)

100 catch up drill

100 finger tip drag drill

6x50 freestyle descend the set
w/:15R

200 freestyle (L3)

200 pull (L3)

100 kick (L5)

100 kick (L2)

100 choice of stroke (L2)

TOTAL: 1600

L1: Recovery; L2: Aerobic; L3: High-End Aerobic to Low Anaerobic;
L4: Lactate or Anaerobic Threshold; L5: Sub-Maximum to Maximum Effort

15
≈≈≈

300 choice of stroke (L2)

100; 25 right arm drill/25 left arm drill/50 freestyle

2x100 kick (L2) w/:10R

4x50 catch-up drill w/:10R

2x50 finger tip drag drill w/:10R

2x100 freestyle (L4) w/:15R

100 freestyle (L5)

2x100 pull (L4) w/:15R

200 choice of stroke (L2)

TOTAL: 1600

L1: Recovery; L2: Aerobic; L3: High-End Aerobic to Low Anaerobic;
L4: Lactate or Anaerobic Threshold; L5: Sub-Maximum to Maximum Effort

16

≋

200 choice of stroke (L2)
300 pull (L3)

4x50 6-3-6 drill w/:10R
2x50 finger tip drag drill w/:10R

8x75 freestyle build each w/:10R
100; 50 backstroke/50 breaststroke
(L3)

100 choice of stroke (L2)

TOTAL: 1600

17
≈≈≈

200 choice of stroke (L2)

4x50; 25 kick on back no board/25 stroke your choice (L2) w/:10R

4x100 freestyle build each w/:25R

2x200 pull build each w/:20R

100 kick (L2)

300 choice of stroke (L2)

TOTAL: 1600

18

200 choice of stroke (L2)

250 pull (L3)

3x50 kick; 25 flutter/25 your choice (L2) w/:10R

3x100; 25 right arm drill/25 left arm drill/50 freestyle w/:15R

4x75; 25 butterfly/25 backstroke/25 breaststroke (L3) w/:10R

8x25 freestyle (L5) w/:10R

100 kick (L4)

200 choice of stroke (L2)

TOTAL: 1700

L1: Recovery; **L2**: Aerobic; **L3**: High-End Aerobic to Low Anaerobic;
L4: Lactate or Anaerobic Threshold; **L5**: Sub-Maximum to Maximum Effort

19

300 choice of stroke (L2)

2x100; 50 catch up drill/50 fist drill
w/:10R

5x100 freestyle (L4) w/:30R

2x100 pull (L4) w/:10R

2x200 freestyle (L3) w/:20R

200 choice of stroke (L2)

TOTAL: 1800

L1: Recovery; L2: Aerobic; L3: High-End Aerobic to Low Anaerobic;
L4: Lactate or Anaerobic Threshold; L5: Sub-Maximum to Maximum Effort

20

300 choice of stroke (L2)

300 pull (L3)

2x100 kick (L3) w/:10R

4x50 6-3-6 drill w/:10R

2x50 finger tip drag drill w/:10R

6x75 freestyle (L4) w/:10R

150; 50 freestyle/50 breaststroke/50 freestyle (L4) w/:20R

100 choice of stroke (L2)

TOTAL: 1800

L1: Recovery; L2: Aerobic; L3: High-End Aerobic to Low Anaerobic;
L4: Lactate or Anaerobic Threshold; L5: Sub-Maximum to Maximum Effort

21

100 choice of stroke (L2)

100 catch up drill
6x50 kick (L3) w/:10R

500 freestyle; 300 (L3)/200 (L5)
2x300 pull (L4) w/:40R

200 choice of stroke (L2)

TOTAL: 1800

L1: Recovery; L2: Aerobic; L3: High-End Aerobic to Low Anaerobic;
L4: Lactate or Anaerobic Threshold; L5: Sub-Maximum to Maximum Effort

22

200 choice of stroke (L2)

100 6-3-6 drill

3x100; 25 right arm drill/25 left arm drill/50 freestyle w/:10R

2x200 pull (L3) w/:20R

2x50 kick (L2) w/:10R

5x100 freestyle (L4) w/:15R

4x25 freestyle (L5) w/:15R

200 choice of stroke (L2)

TOTAL: 1900

L1: Recovery; **L2**: Aerobic; **L3**: High-End Aerobic to Low Anaerobic;
L4: Lactate or Anaerobic Threshold; **L5**: Sub-Maximum to Maximum Effort

23

≋

200 choice of stroke (L2)

6x50 kick; 25 flutter/25 your choice (L2) w/:10R

300 freestyle locomotion

100, 4x50, 100 freestyle (L5) w/:30R

150, 200, 200, 150; freestyle w/second 50 breaststroke (L3) w/:30R

100 choice of stroke (L2)

TOTAL: 2000

L1: Recovery; **L2**: Aerobic; **L3**: High-End Aerobic to Low Anaerobic;
L4: Lactate or Anaerobic Threshold; **L5**: Sub-Maximum to Maximum Effort

24

≈≈≈

200 choice of stroke (L2)

4x50 kick (L2) w/:10R

4x50 catch up drill w/:10R

2x50 finger tip drag drill w/:10R

3x200 pull (L3) w/:20R

4x50 freestyle descend the set
w/:20R

4x100 freestyle build each w/:15R

100 choice of stroke (L2)

TOTAL: 2000

L1: Recovery; L2: Aerobic; L3: High-End Aerobic to Low Anaerobic;
L4: Lactate or Anaerobic Threshold; L5: Sub-Maximum to Maximum Effort

25

≈≈≈

200 choice of stroke (L2)
2x100 kick (L2) w/:10R

3x100 freestyle (L4) w/:20R
2x200 pull (L2) w/:20R
300 (L4), 200 (L5) freestyle w/:20R

2x50; 25 fist drill/25 freestyle w/:10R
100 6-3-6 drill

100 catch up drill

100 choice of stroke (L2)

TOTAL: 2000

L1: Recovery; **L2**: Aerobic; **L3**: High-End Aerobic to Low Anaerobic;
L4: Lactate or Anaerobic Threshold; **L5**: Sub-Maximum to Maximum Effort

Swim Workouts: 2000-3000 Yards or Meters

NOTE: The distances of these swim workouts reference either meters or yards, whichever is relevant to the pool you use.

1

100 choice of stroke (L2)

100 catch up drill

2x100; 25 right arm drill/25 left arm drill/50 freestyle w/:10R

300 pull (L3)

8x75 freestyle w/:20R;

   descend 1-4

   descend 5-8

2x100 kick; 50 (L3)/50 (L4) w/:10R

2x150; 50 freestyle/50 backstroke/50 freestyle (L3) w/:20R

200 choice of stroke (L2) COOL-DOWN

TOTAL: 2000

2

400 choice of stroke (L2)

200 kick (L2)
4x50 6-3-6 drill w/:10R

4x100 freestyle (L4) w/:15R
2x200 pull (L3) w/:20R

2x100 catch-up drill w/:20R

200 choice of stroke (L2)

TOTAL: 2000

L1: Recovery; **L2**: Aerobic; **L3**: High-End Aerobic to Low Anaerobic;
L4: Lactate or Anaerobic Threshold; **L5**: Sub-Maximum to Maximum Effort

3

≈≈≈

300 choice of stroke (L2)

2x150 pull (L3) w/:15R

5x100 freestyle build each w/:15R

8x75 w/:10R;

  1-4 freestyle (L4)

  **5-8 25 butterfly/25 backstroke/
    25 breaststroke (L3)**

8x25 freestyle (L5) w/:10R

2x100 kick (L2) w/:10R

100 choice of stroke (L2)

TOTAL: 2200

L1: Recovery; L2: Aerobic; L3: High-End Aerobic to Low Anaerobic;
L4: Lactate or Anaerobic Threshold; L5: Sub-Maximum to Maximum Effort

4

200 choice of stroke (L2)

2x50 kick (L2) w/:10R

4x50; 25 catch up drill/25 6-3-6 drill w/:10R

400, 100, 400 freestyle (L4) w/:40R

2x300 pull (L3) w/:20R

100 kick (L3)

100 choice of stroke (L2)

TOTAL: 2200

L1: Recovery; L2: Aerobic; L3: High-End Aerobic to Low Anaerobic;
L4: Lactate or Anaerobic Threshold; L5: Sub-Maximum to Maximum Effort

5

300 choice of stroke (L2)

2x200 pull (L3) w/:20R

4x50 6-3-6 drill w/:10R

4x50 catch-up drill w/:10R

250 pull (L3) w/:15R

2x200 freestyle (L5) broken at the 100 for :05R w/:20R

10x25 freestyle (L4) w/:10R

200 choice of stroke (L2)

TOTAL: 2200

L1: Recovery; L2: Aerobic; L3: High-End Aerobic to Low Anaerobic;
L4: Lactate or Anaerobic Threshold; L5: Sub-Maximum to Maximum Effort

6

300 choice of stroke (L2)

100; 25 right arm drill/25 left arm drill/50 freestyle w/:10R

2x100 kick (L2) w/:10R

5x100 freestyle (L4) w/:30R

2x150 pull (L4) w/:20R

2x200 freestyle (L3) w/:30R

200 pull (L3)

200 choice of stroke (L2)

TOTAL: 2200

L1: Recovery; L2: Aerobic; L3: High-End Aerobic to Low Anaerobic;
L4: Lactate or Anaerobic Threshold; L5: Sub-Maximum to Maximum Effort

7

100 choice of stroke (L2)

2x300 pull (L3) w/:30R

8x75 freestyle (L4) w/:20R

3x150 freestyle; 50 (L3)/50 build/ 50 (L4) w/:20R

2x150 freestyle (L5) w/:30R

3x50 kick (L5) w/:10R

200 choice of stroke (L2)

TOTAL: 2400

L1: Recovery; L2: Aerobic; L3: High-End Aerobic to Low Anaerobic;
L4: Lactate or Anaerobic Threshold; L5: Sub-Maximum to Maximum Effort

8
≈≈≈

200 choice of stroke (L2)

4x50 kick (L2) w/:10R

3x100; 25 right arm drill/25 left arm drill/50 freestyle w/:20R

3x100, 300 pull (L4) w/:30R

400 freestyle (L4)

150, 200, 150; 1st 50 freestyle/2nd 50 freestyle/the rest choice of stroke (L4) w/:30R

200 freestyle (L2)

TOTAL: 2400

L1: Recovery; L2: Aerobic; L3: High-End Aerobic to Low Anaerobic;
L4: Lactate or Anaerobic Threshold; L5: Sub-Maximum to Maximum Effort

9

300 choice of stroke (L2)

4x50 6-3-6 drill w/:15R

4x50 kick (L2) w/:15R

2x100; 25 right arm drill/25 left arm drill/50 freestyle (L2) w/:15R

2x200 pull (L3) w/:20R

4x100 freestyle descend the set w/:15R

6x75 freestyle (L5) w/:15R

4x25 IM order (L3) w/:10R

150 choice of stroke (L2)

TOTAL: 2400

L1: Recovery; **L2**: Aerobic; **L3**: High-End Aerobic to Low Anaerobic;
L4: Lactate or Anaerobic Threshold; **L5**: Sub-Maximum to Maximum Effort

10

300 choice of stroke (L2)

3x100 kick (L2) w/:10R

3x100 freestyle (L4) w/:20R
500 pull (L3)

2x:
  4x50 freestyle (L5) w/:20R
  200 pull (L3)

200 freestyle (L2)

TOTAL: 2400

L1: Recovery; L2: Aerobic; L3: High-End Aerobic to Low Anaerobic;
L4: Lactate or Anaerobic Threshold; L5: Sub-Maximum to Maximum Effort

11

350 choice of stroke (L2)

3x100; 25 head up drill/75 freestyle
   w/:15R

300 pull (L3)
10x75 freestyle w/:20R;
   1-5 (L4)
   6-10 (L5)
3x150; 50 freestyle/50 stroke your
   choice/50 freestyle (L3) w/:20R

250 freestyle (L2)

TOTAL: 2400

L1: Recovery; L2: Aerobic; L3: High-End Aerobic to Low Anaerobic;
L4: Lactate or Anaerobic Threshold; L5: Sub-Maximum to Maximum Effort

12

200 choice of stroke (L2)

4x50 catch up drill w/:10R
4x50 kick (L3) w/:10R

7x100 freestyle (L4) w/:30R
3x200 pull (L3) w/:30R
4x50 kick (L5) w/:10R

300 choice of stroke (L2)

TOTAL: 2400

13

400 choice of stroke (L2)

5x50; 25 finger tip drag drill/25 6-3-6 drill w/:10R

5x50 kick (L2) w/:10R

5x100 freestyle build each w/:15R

3x200 pull (L3) w/:20R

200 kick (L2)

200 choice of stroke (L2)

TOTAL: 2400

L1: Recovery; **L2**: Aerobic; **L3**: High-End Aerobic to Low Anaerobic;
L4: Lactate or Anaerobic Threshold; **L5**: Sub-Maximum to Maximum Effort

14
≋

300 choice of stroke (L2)

150 pull (L3)

5x100; 25 right arm drill/25 left arm
    drill/50 freestyle w/:15R

6x50 kick (L3) w/:10R

8x75 w/:20R;

   1-4 freestyle (L5)

   5-8 IM order by 25 (L4)

3x150 freestyle (L4) w/:20R

8x25 freestyle (L5) w/:10R

100 choice of stroke (L2)

TOTAL: 2600

L1: Recovery; L2: Aerobic; L3: High-End Aerobic to Low Anaerobic;
L4: Lactate or Anaerobic Threshold; L5: Sub-Maximum to Maximum Effort

15

300 choice of stroke (L2)
5x50 kick w/:10R (L2)

500 freestyle (L4)
2x300 pull (L3) w/:30R

200 kick (L3)
2x50, 75, 100, 75, 2x50 freestyle (L4)
w/:20R

100 kick (L5)

200 choice of stroke (L2)

TOTAL: 2600

L1: Recovery; L2: Aerobic; L3: High-End Aerobic to Low Anaerobic;
L4: Lactate or Anaerobic Threshold; L5: Sub-Maximum to Maximum Effort

16

≋

300 choice of stroke (L2)

4x50 catch up drill

2x100; 25 right arm drill/25 left arm drill/50 freestyle w/:15R

2x200 pull (L3) w/:30R

6x50 kick (L2) w/:10R

100, 200, 300, 200 freestyle (L4) w/:30R

10x25 freestyle (L5) w/:10R

150 choice of stroke (L2)

TOTAL: 2600

L1: Recovery; L2: Aerobic; L3: High-End Aerobic to Low Anaerobic;
L4: Lactate or Anaerobic Threshold; L5: Sub-Maximum to Maximum Effort

17

≈≈≈

200 choice of stroke (L2)
6x50 kick (L2) w/:10R

2x500 freestyle (L4) 1:30R
2x300 pull (L3) w/:40R
100 freestyle (L5)

200 kick (L2)

200 choice of stroke (L2)

TOTAL: 2600

L1: Recovery; **L2**: Aerobic; **L3**: High-End Aerobic to Low Anaerobic;
L4: Lactate or Anaerobic Threshold; **L5**: Sub-Maximum to Maximum Effort

18
≈≈≈

200 choice of stroke (L2)

100 catch up drill

3x100 kick (L2) w/:20R

5x100 freestyle (L4) w/:10R

2x200 freestyle (L3) w/:20R

100, 200, 300, 200, 100 pull (L4) w/:30R

200 choice of stroke (L2)

TOTAL: 2600

19

300 choice of stroke (L2)

2x100; 50 catch up drill/50 finger tip
drag drill w/:10R

3x100, 300 pull (L3) w/:30R

8x75 freestyle (L4) w/:10R

6x150 w/:30R;

1-3 50 freestyle/50 breaststroke/
50 freestyle (L4)

4-6 50 freestyle/50 backstroke/
50 freestyle (L4)

200 choice of stroke (L2)

TOTAL: 2800

L1: Recovery; L2: Aerobic; L3: High-End Aerobic to Low Anaerobic;
L4: Lactate or Anaerobic Threshold; L5: Sub-Maximum to Maximum Effort

20

400 choice of stroke (L2)

4x50 6-3-6 drill w/:10R

4x50 catch up drill w/:10R

4x50 kick (L2) w/:10R

7x100 freestyle (L4) w/:20R

3x200 pull (L4) w/:40R

200 kick (L2)

300 choice of stroke (L2)

TOTAL: 2800

21

300 choice of stroke (L2)

4x100; 25 right arm drill/25 left arm drill/50 freestyle (L2) w/:15R

3x100; 25 head up freestyle/75 freestyle w/:15R

150 pull (L3)

6x50 kick (L2) w/:10R

8x75 freestyle (L4) w/:10R

3x150 freestyle; 50 (L4)/50 (L3)/ 50 (L5) w/:20R

8x25 IM order by 25 (L4) w/:10R

100 choice of stroke (L2)

TOTAL: 2800

L1: Recovery; L2: Aerobic; L3: High-End Aerobic to Low Anaerobic;
L4: Lactate or Anaerobic Threshold; L5: Sub-Maximum to Maximum Effort

22

≋

200 choice of stroke (L2)

4x50 catch up drill w/:20R

6x50 freestyle (L3) w/:10R

2x500 freestyle (L4) w/1:00R

2x300 pull (L3) w/:30R

200 kick (L5)

300 choice of stroke (L2)

TOTAL: 2800

L1: Recovery; L2: Aerobic; L3: High-End Aerobic to Low Anaerobic;
L4: Lactate or Anaerobic Threshold; L5: Sub-Maximum to Maximum Effort

23

300 choice of stroke (L2)

2x100; 50 6-3-6 drill/50 freestyle w/:15R

4x100; 25 right arm drill/25 left arm drill/50 freestyle w/:15R

2x200 pull (L3) w/:30R

6x50; 25 backstroke/25 breaststroke (L4) w/:15R

8x100 freestyle w/:20R;
  1-4 (L3)
  5-8 (L4)

2x100 IM (L3) w/:20R

10x25 freestyle (L5) w/:10R

150 choice of stroke (L2)

TOTAL: 3000

L1: Recovery; **L2**: Aerobic; **L3**: High-End Aerobic to Low Anaerobic;
L4: Lactate or Anaerobic Threshold; **L5**: Sub-Maximum to Maximum Effort

24

300 choice of stroke (L2)

2x200 pull w/:20R (L3)

2x100; 50 catch up drill/50 freestyle w/:15R

4x100; 25 right arm drill/25 left arm drill/50 freestyle w/:10R

6x50 kick (L3) w/:10R

100 freestyle, 150 kick, 200 freestyle, 150 kick, 100 freestyle (L4) w/:30R

3x100 pull (L3) w/:30R

8x25 freestyle (L5) w/:15R

50 kick (L5)

150 choice of stroke (L2)

TOTAL: 3000

L1: Recovery; L2: Aerobic; L3: High-End Aerobic to Low Anaerobic;
L4: Lactate or Anaerobic Threshold; L5: Sub-Maximum to Maximum Effort

25

200 choice of stroke (L2)

2x100; 50 6-3-6 drill/50 freestyle
w/:15R

3x50; 50 catch up drill/50 freestyle
w/:15R (L2)

3x50; 50 finger tip drag drill/
50 freestyle w/:15R (L2)

5x200 freestyle (L4) w/:15R

10x50 freestyle (L4) w/:30R

150, 200, 200, 150 pull (L4) w/:40R

100 choice of stroke (L2)

TOTAL: 3000

L1: Recovery; L2: Aerobic; L3: High-End Aerobic to Low Anaerobic;
L4: Lactate or Anaerobic Threshold; L5: Sub-Maximum to Maximum Effort

Swim Workouts: 3000-4000 Yards or Meters

NOTE: The distances of these swim workouts reference either meters or yards, whichever is relevant to the pool you use.

1

2x150 pull (L3) w/:15R

2x100 kick (L2) w/:15R

5x50; 25 catch up drill/25 freestyle w/:10R

5x50; 25 finger tip drag drill/ 25 freestyle w/:10R

3x100; 25 right arm drill/25 left arm drill/50 freestyle w/:15R

8x75 freestyle descend the set w/:15R

3x150 freestyle (L5) w/:25R

8x25 IM order by 25 (L4) w/:10R

L1: Recovery; L2: Aerobic; L3: High-End Aerobic to Low Anaerobic;
L4: Lactate or Anaerobic Threshold; L5: Sub-Maximum to Maximum Effort

100 kick (L2)
100 choice of stroke (L2)   COOL-DOWN

TOTAL: 3000

2

≋

200 choice of stroke (L2)

2x100; 50 fist drill/50 freestyle
w/:15R

3x100; 25 backstroke/25
breaststroke/50 freestyle (L5)
w/:15R

500, 200, 500 freestyle (L4) w/:45R

300 pull (L3) w/:30R

50, 100, 100, 50 freestyle (L5) w/:20R

200 kick (L3)

300 choice of stroke (L2)

TOTAL: 3000

L1: Recovery; L2: Aerobic; L3: High-End Aerobic to Low Anaerobic;
L4: Lactate or Anaerobic Threshold; L5: Sub-Maximum to Maximum Effort

3

≋

400 choice of stroke (L2)

150 kick (L2)

150 pull (L2)

4x25 catch up drill w/:10R

8x50 IM order by 25 (L3) w/:10R

5x100 freestyle (L5) w/:30R

200, 2x100 pull; breathe every 3rd stroke (L3) w/:15R

3x200 freestyle (L4) w/1:00R

200 kick (L2)

300 choice of stroke (L2)

TOTAL: 3200

L1: Recovery; L2: Aerobic; L3: High-End Aerobic to Low Anaerobic;
L4: Lactate or Anaerobic Threshold; L5: Sub-Maximum to Maximum Effort

4

~~~

300 choice of stroke (L2)

150 kick (L3)

8x25 6-3-6 drill w/:10R

2x100 catch up drill w/:10R

6x50 freestyle descend the set w/:10R

4x100; 50 freestyle (L5)/50 freestyle (L3) w/:15R

8x75 freestyle (L4) w/:15R

100 kick, 200 pull (L3) w/:20R

3x150 freestyle (L4) w/:20R

L1: Recovery; L2: Aerobic; L3: High-End Aerobic to Low Anaerobic;
L4: Lactate or Anaerobic Threshold; L5: Sub-Maximum to Maximum Effort

8x25 6-3-6 drill w/:10R

100 choice of stroke (L2)

TOTAL: 3200

5

300 choice of stroke (L3)

6x50 w/:10R;
   1-3 catch up drill
   4-6 fist drill
3x100; 25 right arm drill/25 left arm
      drill/50 freestyle w/:15R

2x200 pull build each w/:20R
2x100 freestyle (L5) w/:20R

2x w/:20R:
   4x50 freestyle (L5)
   4x100 (L4)
      1-2 pull
      3-4 freestyle

L1: Recovery; L2: Aerobic; L3: High-End Aerobic to Low Anaerobic;
L4: Lactate or Anaerobic Threshold; L5: Sub-Maximum to Maximum Effort

4x75 kick (L5) w/:25R

100; 50 backstroke/50 breaststroke
    (L2)

100 kick (L2)
 100 choice of stroke (L2)

TOTAL: 3300

6

300 choice of stroke (L2)

100 kick (L2)

200 pull (L2)

4x25 head up freestyle (L2) w/:10R

4x25 catch up drill (L2) w/:10R

6x50 freestyle build each w/:10R

4x75; 25 right arm drill/25 left arm drill/50 freestyle w/:10R

3x100 freestyle build each w/:10R

4x:

100 freestyle (L5) w/:10R

100 your choice stroke or kick (L2)

1:00R between each set

L1: Recovery; L2: Aerobic; L3: High-End Aerobic to Low Anaerobic;
L4: Lactate or Anaerobic Threshold; L5: Sub-Maximum to Maximum Effort

200 kick (L2)

4x:

50 freestyle (L5) w/:10R
50 your choice stroke or kick (L2)
:30R between each set

100 kick (L2)
100 choice of stroke (L2)

TOTAL: 3300

7

≈≈≈

300 choice of stroke (L2)

200 kick (L2)
200 pull (L2)

8x25 alternating; catch up drill/fist drill w/:10
2x150 pull; 25 (L5)/25 (L2)/50 (L5)/50 (L2) w/:25R

4x100; 50 kick/50 freestyle (L5) w/:25
6x75; 25 breaststroke (L3)/50 stroke count w/:15
8x50; 25 freestyle (L4)/25 backstroke (L2) w/:15
12x25 freestyle (L5) w/:10

L1: Recovery; L2: Aerobic; L3: High-End Aerobic to Low Anaerobic;
L4: Lactate or Anaerobic Threshold; L5: Sub-Maximum to Maximum Effort

2x w/:20R:

100 IM (L4)

75; 25 breaststroke/50 freestyle (L3)

50 freestyle (L4)

25 kick on your back (no board) (L2)

150 choice of stroke (L2)

TOTAL: 3400

8

300 choice of stroke (L2)

4x100; 25 right arm drill/25 left arm drill/50 freestyle w/:15R

8x25 alternate; head up drill/6-3-6 drill w/:15R

2x200 pull (L3) w/:20R

6x50 freestyle descend the set w/:10R

300 pull locomotion

5x100 freestyle (L5) w/:15R

500 pull locomotion

10x25 freestyle (L4) w/:10R

250 choice of stroke (L2)

TOTAL: 3400

L1: Recovery; L2: Aerobic; L3: High-End Aerobic to Low Anaerobic;
L4: Lactate or Anaerobic Threshold; L5: Sub-Maximum to Maximum Effort

9

300 choice of stroke (L2)

4x50; 25 fist drill/25 stroke count w/:10R

100 6-3-6 drill

2x300 freestyle build each w/:30R

2x250 pull (L4) w/:30R

4x100; 50 backstroke/50 freestyle (L3) w/:20R

150, 200, 200, 150; every second 50 different stroke than freestyle (L4) w/:30R

12x25 freestyle (L5) w/:15R

[Continued on next page]

150 kick (L2)
150 choice of stroke (L2)

TOTAL: 3400

10

300 choice of stroke (L2)

4x25 alternate; right arm drill/left arm drill w/:10R

4x25 kick on back, no board w/:10R

4x25 stroke count w/:10R

300 freestyle locomotion

2x200 freestyle (L4) w/:30R

2x:

   4x50 pull (L4) w/:15R

   2x100 freestyle (L4) w/:20R

   4x50 kick (L5) w/:15R

100 IM (L3)

6x75 freestyle (L4) w/:20R

[Continued on next page]

100 IM (L3)

4x25 freestyle (L5) w/:10R

100 kick (L4)

150 choice of stroke (L2)

TOTAL: 3500

11

~~~

300 choice of stroke (L2)

100 pull (L2)

150 kick (L2)

6x50 w/:10R;

    1-3 catch up drill

    4-6 fist drill

100; 50 catch up/50 6-3-6 drill

**6x50 freestyle descend the set
    w/:10R**

2x500 w/1:00R;

    1 freestyle (L3)

    2 pull locomotion

300; 100 IM/200 freestyle (L3)

200 pull (L3)

[Continued on next page]

2x50, 75, 100, 75, 2x50 freestyle (L4) w/:25R

100 kick (L2)
200 choice of stroke (L2)

TOTAL: 3500

12

300 choice of stroke (L2)

200 kick (L2)

200 pull (L2)

4x75; 25 finger tip drag drill/50 stroke count w/:15R

2x100; 50 butterfly-backstroke/ 50 free (L3) w/:15R

3x50 freestyle (L5) w/:10R

2x100; 25 breaststroke/75 freestyle (L3) w/:15R

4x75; 25 catch-up drill/50 stroke count w/:10R

3x:

4x25 IM order by 25 (L3) w/:10R

4x25 freestyle (L5) w/:15R

[Continued on next page]

4x25 pull (L3) w/:15R

150 kick (L2)

100 freestyle (L5)

100 kick (L2)

100 choice of stroke (L2)

TOTAL: 3500

13

400 choice of stroke (L2)

200 kick (L2)

4x75; 25 right arm drill/25 left arm drill/25 freestyle w/:15R

150 kick (L2)

4x75; 25 freestyle/25 finger tip drag drill/25 freestyle w/:15R

50 fist drill

100 freestyle (L5)

150; 50 freestyle/50 6-3-6 drill/ 50 freestyle (L2)

200 pull (L3)

250 freestyle (L5)

200 pull (L3)

[Continued on next page]

**150; 50 freestyle/50 6-3-6 drill/
   50 freestyle (L2)**

100 freestyle (L5)

50 fist drill

2x w/:20R:

   100 IM (L3)

   50 kick (L2)

   100 freestyle (L5)

   50 kick (L2)

100 freestyle (L4)

2x50 kick (L5) w/:15R

100 kick (L2)

100 choice of stroke (L2)

TOTAL: 3600

L1: Recovery; L2: Aerobic; L3: High-End Aerobic to Low Anaerobic;
L4: Lactate or Anaerobic Threshold; L5: Sub-Maximum to Maximum Effort

14

300 choice of stroke (L2)

100; 50 catch up drill/50 6-3-6 drill

4x100; 25 right arm drill/25 left arm drill/50 freestyle w/:10R

2x200 pull (L3) w/:30R

6x50 freestyle descend the set w/:10R

100 pull, 200 freestyle, 300 pull, 200 freestyle, 100 pull (L4) w/:30R

6x100 freestyle fastest average w/:40R

10x25 IM order by 25 (L3) w/:10R

[Continued on next page]

100 kick (L2)

250 choice of stroke (L2)

TOTAL: 3600

15

200 freestyle (L2)

100 kick (L2)

100 kick no board (L2)

200 pull (L2)

4x25 6-3-6 drill w/:10R

3x150; 25 right arm drill/25 left arm drill/100 freestyle w/:20R

4x25 6-3-6 drill w/:10R

3x50 freestyle (L3) w/:10R

4x100 kick; 50 flutter (L4)/ 50 back-breast (L2) w/:10R

3x50 freestyle (L3) w/:10R

2x150 freestyle (L5) w/:30R

2x100 pull (L3) w/:10R

[Continued on next page]

2x:

   100 kick (L4)

   4x50; 25 finger tip drag drill/
      25 6-3-6 drill w/:10R

   :30R between each set

300 pull locomotion

50 freestyle (L5)

100 kick (L2)

100 choice of stroke (L2)

TOTAL: 3600

L1: Recovery; L2: Aerobic; L3: High-End Aerobic to Low Anaerobic;
L4: Lactate or Anaerobic Threshold; L5: Sub-Maximum to Maximum Effort

16

300 freestyle (L2)

200 kick (L2)

200 pull (L2)

3x50 catch-up drill w/:10R

3x50 6-3-6 drill w/:10R

3x50 kick (L4) w/:10R

150 freestyle (L5)

200 pull (L3)

150 kick (L2)

2x100 freestyle (L4) w/:30R

4x75; 25 butterfly/25 backstroke/
    25 breaststroke (L3) w/:20R

6x50 freestyle (L4) w/:20R

8x25 kick (L4) w/:10R

[Continued on next page]

4x125 freestyle build each w/:20R

5x50 freestyle fastest average w/:20R

150 kick (L2)

150 choice of stroke (L2)

TOTAL: 3700

17

200 freestyle (L2)

200 kick (L2)

4x25; odds head up freestyle, evens
     6-3-6 drill w/:10R

2x75; 25 fist drill/50 freestyle w/:10R

6x50 pull; 25 (L3)/25 (L4) w/:15R

5x100 freestyle; 50 (L3)/50 (L4)
     w/:10R

3x:

     4x25 freestyle (L5) w/:10R

     100 your choice (L2)

     1:00R between each set

150 kick (L2)

[Continued on next page]

2x:

> **2x25 freestyle (L5) w/:10R**
>
> **100 your choice (L2)**
>
> **:30R between each set**

4x75; 25 backstroke/25 breaststroke/25 freestyle w/:15R

4x75 kick; 25 dolphin/25 breast/ 25 flutter w/:15R

300 pull locomotion

100 kick (L2)

200 choice of stroke (L2)

TOTAL: 3700

18

300 freestyle (L2)

200 kick (L2)

200 pull (L2)

4x25 freestyle build each w/:10R

3x:

   3x50 w/:10R;

      1 25 catch-up drill/25 kick on back

      2 25 freestyle/25 kick on back

      3 25 pull/25 kick on back

3x100 freestyle fastest average w/:30R

200 pull (L2)

[Continued on next page]

3x100 freestyle fastest average w/:30R

200 kick (L2)

3x100 freestyle fastest average w/:30R

200 alternate; backstroke/ breaststroke by 25

8x25 freestyle; odds (L5), evens (L3) w/:15R

8x25 IM order by 25 w/:15R

8x25 kick (L4) w/:10R

200 alternate; backstroke/ breaststroke by 25

100 kick (L2)

150 choice of stroke (L2)

TOTAL: 3800

L1: Recovery; L2: Aerobic; L3: High-End Aerobic to Low Anaerobic;
L4: Lactate or Anaerobic Threshold; L5: Sub-Maximum to Maximum Effort

19

200 freestyle (L2)

200 kick (L2)

200 pull (L2)

6x25 6-3-6 drill w/:10R

6x75; 25 right arm drill/25 left arm drill/25 catch-up drill w/:15R

6x25 fist drill w/:10R

3x50 freestyle (L4) w/:10R

4x100 kick; 50 flutter (L4)/50 breast (L2) w/:15R

4x50 freestyle build each w/:15R

2x150 freestyle (L5) w/:30R

2x100 pull (L3) w/:20R

2x100 kick (L2) w/:10R

[Continued on next page]

4x50; 25 freestyle/25 breaststroke (L5) w/:10R

300 pull (L4)

2x125 kick; 25 breast (L2)/75 flutter (L4)/25 breast (L2) w/:20R

2x125; 25 breaststroke (L2)/75 freestyle (L4)/25 breaststroke (L2) w/:20R

150 pull (L2)

TOTAL: 3800

L1: Recovery; L2: Aerobic; L3: High-End Aerobic to Low Anaerobic;
L4: Lactate or Anaerobic Threshold; L5: Sub-Maximum to Maximum Effort

20

200 freestyle (L2)

150 kick (L2)

200 pull (L2)

8x25; odds head up freestyle, evens freestyle (L3) w/:10R

4x75; 25 catch up drill/25 finger tip drag drill/25 freestyle w/:15R

6x50 freestyle build each w/:15R

400 freestyle (L4) w/:20R

4x:

75 freestyle (L5) w/:10R

50 your choice freestyle or kick no board (L2)

1:00R between each set

[Continued on next page]

200 kick (L2)

4x:

25 freestyle (L5) w/:10R

25 your choice freestyle or kick no board (L2)

:15R between each set

500 pull (L3)

6x75; 25 backstroke/25 breaststroke/25 freestyle (L3) w/:15R

200 choice of stroke (L2)

TOTAL: 3800

21

150 freestyle (L2)

100 kick (L2)

200 pull (L3)

150 freestyle (L3)

2x150; 50 catch-up drill/
    50 freestyle/50 catch-up drill
    w/:20R

8x25 6-3-6 drill w/:10R

6x25 freestyle alternate; 25 (L3),
    25 (L4), 25 (L3) w/:10R

6x75 pull build each w/:20R

4x100 IM (L3) w/:20R

8x25 kick (L3) w/:10R

[Continued on next page]

8x25 freestyle (L5) w/:10R

8x25 pull (L3) w/:10R

2x500 w/:40R;
　1 freestyle (L4)
　2 alternate; 100 kick no board/
　　100 freestyle (L3)

100 kick (L2)

200 choice of stroke (L2)

TOTAL: 4000

L1: Recovery; L2: Aerobic; L3: High-End Aerobic to Low Anaerobic;
L4: Lactate or Anaerobic Threshold; L5: Sub-Maximum to Maximum Effort

22

300 freestyle (L2)

4x50 kick (L2) w/:10R

2x100 pull (L2) w/:10R

8x50; 25 catch-up drill/25 freestyle w/:10R

4x100 pull descend the set w/:20R

4x125 freestyle; 50 (L5)/75 (L3) w/:20R

200 kick (L3)

2x w/:20R:

50 kick (L4)

100; 25 backstroke/25 freestyle/ 25 backstroke/25 freestyle (L3)

200 freestyle (L5)

[Continued on next page]

100; 25 breaststroke/25 freestyle/
25 breaststroke/25 freestyle (L3)

50 kick (L4)

12x25 freestyle (L5) w/:15R

12x25 IM order by 25 (L3) w/:15R

200 choice of stroke (L2)

TOTAL: 4000

L1: Recovery; L2: Aerobic; L3: High-End Aerobic to Low Anaerobic;
L4: Lactate or Anaerobic Threshold; L5: Sub-Maximum to Maximum Effort

23

300 freestyle (L2)

200 kick (L2)

200 pull (L2)

4x25 6-3-6 drill w/:20R

2x150; 25 right arm drill/25 left arm drill/100 freestyle w/:20R

5x50 freestyle (L5) w/:10R

3x100 kick; 50 flutter/25 breast/ 25 back (L2) w/:15R

3x w/:30R:

   200 freestyle (L4)

   100 choice of stroke (L2)

   200 pull (L3)

   100 freestyle (L5)

[Continued on next page]

4x100 kick (L4) w/:20R

150 choice of stroke (L2)

TOTAL: 4000

24

300 freestyle (L2)

2x100 kick (L2) w/:20R

200 pull (L2)

2x50 catch-up drill w/:15R

6x25 stroke count w/:10R

4x75; 25 6-3-6 drill/25 catch-up drill/ 25 freestyle w/:15R

6x25 stroke count w/:10R

100 lowest stroke count possible

2x100 pull (L2) w/:15R

2x150 freestyle (L5) broken at 100 for :05 w/:25R

2x100 kick (L2) w/:15R

2x150 freestyle (L5) broken at 75 for :05 w/:25R

[Continued on next page]

2x100 your choice on stroke (L2) w/:15R

2x150 freestyle (L4) w/:25R

4x50 kick (L3) w/:15R

4x100 (L3) w/:20R;

   1 IM

   2 freestyle

   3 pull

   4 freestyle

4x50 pull stroke count w/:15R

100 freestyle; 25 (L5)/75 (L2)

100 choice of stroke (L2)

TOTAL: 4000

L1: Recovery; L2: Aerobic; L3: High-End Aerobic to Low Anaerobic;
L4: Lactate or Anaerobic Threshold; L5: Sub-Maximum to Maximum Effort

25

300 choice of stroke (L2)

2x200 pull (L2) w/:20R

6x50 kick (L2) w/:10R

4x100; 25 right arm drill/25 left arm drill/50 freestyle w/:10R

8x100 freestyle w/:20R;

  1-2 freestyle - 1 (L2), 2 (L4)

  3-4 kick - 3 (L2), 4 (L4)

  5-6 pull - 5 (L2), 6 (L4)

  7-8 freestyle (L5)

2x150 pull; 50 breathe every 3rd, 50 breathe every 5th, 50 breathe every 3rd w/:20R

[Continued on next page]

500 freestyle (L4)

10x50 freestyle (L4) w/:15R
12x25 IM order by 25 (L3) w/:10R

200 choice of stroke (L2)

TOTAL: 4000

Swim Workouts: 4000-5000 Yards or Meters

NOTE: The distances of these swim workouts reference either meters or yards, whichever is relevant to the pool you use.

300 freestyle (L2)   WARM-UP

100 kick (L2)

200 pull (L2)

8x25; odds head up freestyle, evens 6-3-6 drill w/:10R

6x50 pull; 25 (L2)/25 (L4) w/:10R

4x75; odds fist drill, evens 25 right arm drill/25 left arm drill/ 25 freestyle w/:10R

3x100 pull; 75 (L2)/25 (L4) w/:20R

4x freestyle:

100 fastest time w/:45R

50 fastest time w/:10R

L1: Recovery; L2: Aerobic; L3: High-End Aerobic to Low Anaerobic;
L4: Lactate or Anaerobic Threshold; L5: Sub-Maximum to Maximum Effort

100 your choice on stroke (L2)

1:00R between each set

150 kick (L2)

300 pull locomotion

6x75; 25 backstroke/25 breaststroke/25 freestyle (L3) w/:20R

4x75 kick; odds 25 dolphin/25 breast/ 25 flutter, evens flutter (L3) w/:20R

100 choice of stroke (L2)   COOL-DOWN

TOTAL: 4000

2

300 freestyle (L2)

100 kick (L2)

200 pull (L2)

6x50; 25 catch-up drill/25 stroke count w/:15R

4x50; 25 fist drill/25 finger tip drag drill w/:15R

4x25 kick (L2) w/:15R

4x25 kick breast (L2) w/:15R

4x25 kick (L2) w/:15R

4x25 kick back (L2) w/:15R

4x75 pull build w/:15R

100 freestyle build w/:15R

L1: Recovery; L2: Aerobic; L3: High-End Aerobic to Low Anaerobic;
L4: Lactate or Anaerobic Threshold; L5: Sub-Maximum to Maximum Effort

50 choice of stroke (L2)

500 pull locomotion

50 choice of stroke (L2)

300 freestyle (L4)

50 choice of stroke (L2)

200 kick (L2)

250 freestyle (L4)

100 pull (L3)

150 freestyle (L5)

50 choice (L2)

150 alternate; 25 butterfly/
    25 backstroke (L3)

50 choice (L2)

100 kick (L2)

100 choice of stroke (L2)

TOTAL: 4000

3

200 freestyle (L2)

100 kick (L2)

200 pull (L2)

8x25; odds your choice on stroke, evens catch-up drill w/:10R

8x25 stroke count w/:10R

3x50 freestyle build each w/:15R

3x50 pull build each w/:15R

2x75 freestyle build each w/:15

2x75 pull build each w/:15R

100 kick (L2)

2x100 kick (L4) w/:20R

50 kick (L5)

L1: Recovery; **L2**: Aerobic; **L3**: High-End Aerobic to Low Anaerobic;
L4: Lactate or Anaerobic Threshold; **L5**: Sub-Maximum to Maximum Effort

100 pull (L3)
2x100 pull (L4) w/:15R
50 pull (L2)

100 freestyle (L2)
2x100 freestyle (L5) w/:20R
50 freestyle (L2)

4x25 IM order (L3) w/:10R
2x100 IM (L4) w/:15R

50 breaststroke (L2)
100 kick (L2)
3x50 kick (L4) w/:15R

50; 25 butterfly/25 backstroke (L3)
3x50 pull (L3) w/:15R
50 freestyle (L2)
3x50 freestyle (L5) w/:15R

[Continued on next page]

50 freestyle (L2)

3x50; 25 butterfly/25 backstroke (L4) w/:20R

50 freestyle (L2)

100 kick (L2)

100 choice of stroke (L2)

TOTAL: 4000

L1: Recovery; L2: Aerobic; L3: High-End Aerobic to Low Anaerobic;
L4: Lactate or Anaerobic Threshold; L5: Sub-Maximum to Maximum Effort

4
≈≈≈

200 freestyle (L2)
200 kick (L2)

200 pull (L2)

4x25 alternate; catch-up drill/fist drill
w/:10R

100 pull (L2)

4x25 alternate; breaststroke/
backstroke w/:10R

100 pull (L2)

4x25 alternate; 6-3-6 drill/finger tip
drag drill w/:10R

100 pull (L2)

2x50 kick (L2) w/:10R

4x75 freestyle (L4) w/:15R

2x100 IM (L3) w/:15R

[Continued on next page]

200 freestyle (L4)

**150; 50 freestyle/50 6-3-6 drill/
50 freestyle (L2)**

200 pull (L3)

200 freestyle (L5)

200 pull (L3)

**150; 50 freestyle/50 6-3-6 drill/
50 freestyle (L2)**

4x100 freestyle (L5) w/:40R

2x50 kick (L2) w/:10R

2x75 freestyle (L5) w/:40R

2x50 kick (L2) w/:10R

6x50 freestyle (L5) w/:40R

2x50 kick (L2) w/:10R

150 choice of stroke (L2)

TOTAL: 4200

L1: Recovery; L2: Aerobic; L3: High-End Aerobic to Low Anaerobic;
L4: Lactate or Anaerobic Threshold; L5: Sub-Maximum to Maximum Effort

5

400 freestyle (L2)

200 kick (L2)

150; 50 finger tip drag drill/50 6-3-6 drill/50 finger tip drag drill w/:15R

2x150 pull (L2) w/:15R

150; 50 6-3-6 drill/50 catch up drill/50 6-3-6 drill w/:15R

4x50 kick (L3) w/:05R

4x75; 25 butterfly/25 backstroke/ 25 breaststroke (L3) w/:20R

4x100 freestyle (L4) w/:20R

200 freestyle (L4)

200 pull (L2)

[Continued on next page]

200 non-freestyle; your choice of stroke (L3)

4x125 freestyle (L4) w/:15

4x50; 25 backstroke/25 breaststroke (L3) w/:05R

500 pull locomotion

100 kick (L2)

200 choice of stroke (L2)

TOTAL: 4200

L1: Recovery; **L2**: Aerobic; **L3**: High-End Aerobic to Low Anaerobic;
L4: Lactate or Anaerobic Threshold; **L5**: Sub-Maximum to Maximum Effort

6

200 freestyle (L2)

200 kick (L2)

200 pull (L2)

8x25 6-3-6 drill w/:10R

8x25 catch-up drill w/:10R

8x25 freestyle descend the set
      w/:10R

6x50; 25 6-3-6 drill/25 kick on back
      (no board) w/:10R

2x:

   3x100; 25 kick on back/25 kick on
      right side/25 kick on left side/
      25 kick on back (L3) w/:15R

   2x150 freestyle (L5) w/:20R

   3x100 pull; breathe every 3rd, 5th,
      7th, 5th stroke by 25 w/:25R

[Continued on next page]

2x freestyle build each w/:15R:
    50
    75
    100
    75
    50

100 kick (L2)
100 choice of stroke (L2)

TOTAL: 4200

7

~~~~~

200 freestyle (L2)

200 kick (L2)

200 pull (L2)

4x25 alternate; catch-up drill/ freestyle w/:05R

4x50; odds 6-3-6 drill, evens freestyle w/:10R

4x75 freestyle; 25 (L4)/50 (L2)

4x100 freestyle; 50 (L4)/50 (L2)

6x25; odds breaststroke, evens freestyle (L3) w/:05R

6x50 kick; 25 (L4)/25 (L2) w/:05R

6x75 w/:20R;

    1-3 IM order (L3)

    4-6 freestyle (L4)

[Continued on next page]

6x100 pull; 50 (L5)/50 (L3) w/:25R

400 freestyle (L4)

w/:10R

  100 kick (L2)

  150 pull (L3)

  100 kick (L5)

  150 pull (L5)

  100 kick (L2)

100 choice of stroke (L2)

TOTAL: 4200

L1: Recovery; L2: Aerobic; L3: High-End Aerobic to Low Anaerobic;
L4: Lactate or Anaerobic Threshold; L5: Sub-Maximum to Maximum Effort

8

200 freestyle (L2)

200 pull (L2)

3x50 kick (L2) w/:10R

2x75 freestyle (L2) w/:10R

3x50 6-3-6 drill w/:10R

2x75 pull (L2) w/:10

4x75; 25 catch-up drill/25 finger tip drag drill/25 fist drill w/:10R

500 pull locomotion

2x200 freestyle broken at the 100 for :05R (L5) w/:40R

100 kick (L2)

3x100 pull broken at the 50 for :05 (L5) w/:15R

[Continued on next page]

100 freestyle (L2)

2x50 freestyle (L5) w/:10R

100 kick (L2)

100 pull broken at the 50 for :05 (L5)

100 pull (L2)

4x25 kick (L3) w/:10R

100 freestyle (L5)

4x25 6-3-6 drill w/:10R

100 pull (L4)

4x25 kick; mix strokes (L2) w/:10R

100 freestyle (L5)

4x100 kick; 50 (L3)/50 (L4) w/:20R

100 choice of stroke (L2)

TOTAL: 4200

L1: Recovery; L2: Aerobic; L3: High-End Aerobic to Low Anaerobic;
L4: Lactate or Anaerobic Threshold; L5: Sub-Maximum to Maximum Effort

9
≈≈≈

300 freestyle (L2)

200 kick (L2)

200 pull (L2)

8x25 catch-up drill w/:10R

3x50 kick (L3) w/:10R

8x25 6-3-6 drill w/:10R

2x150 pull (L3) w/:20R

200 pull (L4)

150 kick (L4)

2x100 freestyle (L5) w/:20R

4x75; 25 but terfly/25 backstroke/
      25 breaststroke (L3) w/:20R

6x50 freestyle (L4) w/:25R

8x25 kick (L4) w/:10R

[Continued on next page]

3x200 freestyle; 50 (L4)/75 (L4)/ 50 (L2)/25 (L4) w/:30R

10x50 freestyle fastest average w/:30R

200 choice of stroke (L2)

TOTAL: 4200

10

300 freestyle (L2)

100 kick (L2)

200 pull (L2)

4x25 6-3-6 drill w/:10R

3x150 w/:25R;

> 1 50 right arm drill/50 left arm drill/50 freestyle
>
> 2 50 butterfly right arm drill/50 butterfly left arm drill/50 butterfly
>
> 3 50 right arm drill/50 left arm drill/50 freestyle

4x25 6-3-6 drill w/:10R

3x50 freestyle descend the set w/:10R

4x100 kick; 50 flutter/50 breast (L3) w/:10R

[Continued on next page]

3x50 freestyle (L4) w/:10R

300 freestyle (L4)

2x:

   2x150 freestyle (L4) w/:30R

   2x100 pull (L3) w/:15R

   100 kick (L5) w/:15R

   4x50; 25 catch-up drill/25 freestyle
      w/:10R

   1:00R between each set

3x100 kick; 25 choice of stroke/
      50 flutter/25 choice of stroke
      (L3) w/:15R

150 pull (L2)
100 choice of stroke (L2)

TOTAL: 4400

L1: Recovery; L2: Aerobic; L3: High-End Aerobic to Low Anaerobic;
L4: Lactate or Anaerobic Threshold; L5: Sub-Maximum to Maximum Effort

11

400 freestyle (L2)

100 kick (L2)

6x100; odds 25 finger tip drag drill/
75 freestyle, evens 25 catch-up
drill/75 freestyle w/:15R

6x50 freestyle w/:10R;

descend 1-3

descend 4-6

2x:

4x50; 25 catch-up drill/25 freestyle
w/:10R

4x50 pull (L2) w/:10R

4x50 freestyle (L5) w/:20R

[Continued on next page]

3x200 freestyle (L4) w/:40R

2x w/:20R:
    50 kick (L4)
    100 pull (L3)
    100 freestyle (L4)
    100 pull (L3)
    50 kick (L4)

12x25 freestyle (L4) w/:10R

100 choice of stroke (L2)

TOTAL: 4400

L1: Recovery; L2: Aerobic; L3: High-End Aerobic to Low Anaerobic;
L4: Lactate or Anaerobic Threshold; L5: Sub-Maximum to Maximum Effort

12

300 freestyle (L2)
200 kick (L2)

200 pull (L2)

50 catch up drill

100 kick (L2)

150 freestyle (L2)

150 pull (L2)

100 kick (L2)

50 catch-up drill

6x25 alternate; finger tip drag
    drill/fist drill w/:10R

200 freestyle; breathe every 3rd (L2)

6x25 alternate; catch-up drill/6-3-6
    drill w/:10R

200 freestyle; breathe every 3rd (L2)

[Continued on next page]

3x w/:30R:
   100 pull (L2)
   100 freestyle (L5)
   100 pull (L2)
   100 IM (L4)

400 pull (L3)

4x50 kick board (L4) w/:10R
2x150; 50 freestyle/50 backstroke/
   50 freestyle (L3) w/:20R
4x50 kick (L3) w/:10R

100 choice of stroke (L2)

TOTAL: 4400

L1: Recovery; L2: Aerobic; L3: High-End Aerobic to Low Anaerobic;
L4: Lactate or Anaerobic Threshold; L5: Sub-Maximum to Maximum Effort

13
~~~~~

300 freestyle (L2)

200 kick (L2)

200 pull (L2)

2x50 catch-up drill w/:10R

6x25 stroke count w/:10R

4x75; 25 6-3-6 drill/25 catch-up drill/25 freestyle w/:10R

6x25 freestyle stroke count w/:10R

100 lowest stroke count possible

2x100 pull (L2) w/:10R

300 freestyle (L5) broken at the 150 for :05R

2x100 kick (L2) w/:15R

300 freestyle (L5) broken at the 100 for :05R

[Continued on next page]

2x100 choice stroke (L2) w/:15R

300 kick (L5) broken at the 150 for :05R

4x50 kick; odds (L4), evens (L2) w/:15R

4x100 (L4) w/:30R;

1 IM

2 freestyle

3 pull

4 freestyle

4x50 pull stroke count w/:10

4x100 freestyle; 25 (L4)/75 (L3) w/:30R

100 kick (L2)

100 choice of stroke (L2)

TOTAL: 4400

L1: Recovery; L2: Aerobic; L3: High-End Aerobic to Low Anaerobic;
L4: Lactate or Anaerobic Threshold; L5: Sub-Maximum to Maximum Effort

14

200 freestyle (L2)

200 kick (L2)

300 pull (L2)

8x50; odds 25 catch-up drill/
25 freestyle, evens 25 fist
drill/25 freestyle w/:15R

4x125; 25 butterfly/75 freestyle/
25 backstroke w/:25R

4x50 freestyle build each w/:15R

2x100 IM (L3) w/:15R

2x125 pull (L3) w/:15R

2x150 freestyle (L4) w/:15R

2x125 pull (L3) w/:15R

2x100 IM (L4) w/:15R

[Continued on next page]

2x200 freestyle (L5) w/:40R

100 kick (L2)

4x50 freestyle build each w/:15R

4x125 kick; 25 breast/75 flutter/ 25 breast (L3) w/:15R

3x100 pull (L3) w/:20R

100 choice of stroke (L2)

TOTAL: 4600

L1: Recovery; L2: Aerobic; L3: High-End Aerobic to Low Anaerobic;
L4: Lactate or Anaerobic Threshold; L5: Sub-Maximum to Maximum Effort

15

300 freestyle (L2)

200 kick (L2)

200 pull (L2)

4x50; 25 6-3-6 drill/25 freestyle
    w/:10R

3x150; 50 backstroke/100 freestyle
    (L3) w/:15R

2x100 freestyle (L4) w/:25R

300 alternate; 50 breaststroke/
    100 freestyle (L3)

2x100 freestyle (L5) w/:15R

5x50; 25 breaststroke/25 freestyle
    (L3) w/:15R

2x100 freestyle (L4) w/:15R

[Continued on next page]

500 freestyle locomotion
100, 4x50, 100 freestyle (L4) w/:20R

100 kick (L2)

8x75 freestyle w/:15R;
   1-4 50 (L3)/25 (L4)
   5-8 50 (L4)/25 (L3)
8x50 pull w/:15R;
   1-4 breathe every 3rd stroke
   5-8 breathe every 5th stroke

100 choice of stroke (L2)

TOTAL: 4600

L1: Recovery; L2: Aerobic; L3: High-End Aerobic to Low Anaerobic;
L4: Lactate or Anaerobic Threshold; L5: Sub-Maximum to Maximum Effort

16

300 freestyle (L2)

200 kick (L2)

200 pull (L2)

6x50; 25 catch-up drill/25 freestyle w/:15R

6x50; 25 6-3-6 drill/25 kick on back (L3) w/:10R

3x100 kick; 50 flutter/50 stroke your choice (L3) w/:20R

2x150 freestyle build each w/:20R

3x100 pull; 50 breathe every 3rd stroke/50 breathe every 5th stroke (L3) w/:15R

200 freestyle (L4)

[Continued on next page]

2x:

3x200 freestyle; 50 (L4)/150 (L3) w/:25R

6x75 kick; 25 flutter (L4)/25 stroke your choice (L2)/25 flutter (L4) w/:15R

100 choice of stroke (L2)

TOTAL: 4600

L1: Recovery; L2: Aerobic; L3: High-End Aerobic to Low Anaerobic;
L4: Lactate or Anaerobic Threshold; L5: Sub-Maximum to Maximum Effort

17

300 freestyle (L2)

200 kick (L2)

200 pull (L2)

4x25 kick your choice of stroke w/:15R

4x25 kick w/:15R

6x50; 25 catch-up drill/25 stroke count w/:15R

4x25 6-3-6 drill w/:15R

4x25 head up drill w/:15R

4x75 pull build each w/:15R

3x100 kick (L4) w/:15R

50 freestyle (L2)

300 pull locomotion

50 freestyle (L4)

[Continued on next page]

3x100 freestyle (L5) w/:30R

50 kick (L2)

3x100 IM (L3) w/:15R

50 freestyle (L2)

200 kick (L2)

400 freestyle alternate; 100 (L4)/
    100 (L2)

2x50 kick; 25 (L4)/25 (L2) w/:15R

50 choice on stroke (L2)

100 pull (L4)

50 choice on stroke (L2)

2x50 freestyle (L5) w/:15R

50 choice on stroke (L2)

2x50; 25 butterfly/25 backstroke (L4)
    w/:15R

L1: Recovery; L2: Aerobic; L3: High-End Aerobic to Low Anaerobic;
L4: Lactate or Anaerobic Threshold; L5: Sub-Maximum to Maximum Effort

50 choice on stroke (L2)

200 kick (L2)

100 choice of stroke (L2)

TOTAL: 4600

18

300 freestyle (L2)

200 kick (L2)

200 pull (L2)

4x100; 25 right arm drill/25 left arm drill/50 freestyle w/:15R

8x50 freestyle descend the set w/:10R

6x150 freestyle w/:25R:

   1-2 50 (L4)/100 (L2)

   3-4 50 (L2)/50 (L4)/50 (L2)

   5-6 50 (L4)/50 (L2)/50 (L4)

1000 freestyle; 200 (L2)/300 (L3)/ 200 (L4)/ 300 (L5)

L1: Recovery; L2: Aerobic; L3: High-End Aerobic to Low Anaerobic;
L4: Lactate or Anaerobic Threshold; L5: Sub-Maximum to Maximum Effort

2x w/:20R:

    50 backstroke (L2)

    100 pull (L3)

    200 freestyle (L5)

    100 pull (L3)

    50 backstroke (L2)

12x25 freestyle (L4) w/:10R

100 choice of stroke (L2)

TOTAL: 4800

19

300 freestyle (L2)
200 kick (L2)

200 pull (L2)

8x25; odds your choice on stroke, evens catch-up drill w/:10R

3x50 freestyle build each w/:05R

3x50 pull build each w/:05R

8x25; odds choice on stroke, evens catch-up drill w/:10R

2x75 freestyle build each w/:10R

2x75 pull build each w/:10R

100 kick (L2)
300 pull (L3)

L1: Recovery; L2: Aerobic; L3: High-End Aerobic to Low Anaerobic;
L4: Lactate or Anaerobic Threshold; L5: Sub-Maximum to Maximum Effort

2x100 freestyle (L4) w/:15R

50 pull (L2)

300 freestyle (L4)

100 IM (L2)

200 IM (L4)

500 freestyle fastest time

50 freestyle (L2)

3x50 kick (L3) w/:20R

150 pull (L3)

150 freestyle (L3)

50 kick (L2)

150; 25 butterfly/25 backstroke/
    100 freestyle (L3)

400 freestyle fastest time

[Continued on next page]

150 kick (L2)

100 choice of stroke (L2)

TOTAL: 4800

20

400 freestyle (L2)

200 kick (L2)

6x50; 25 6-3-6 drill/25 kick on back
     w/:10R

3x100; 50 stroke your choice/
     50 freestyle (L2) w/:10R

2x150; 50 freestyle/50 catch-up
     drill/50 freestyle w/:20R

4x125 freestyle; odds 50 (L4)/
     75 (L3), evens 75 (L2)/50 (L4)
     w/:20R

6x50 kick (L3) w/:15R

4x125 freestyle; odds 100 (L4)/
     25 (L3), evens 75 (L4)/50 (L2)
     w/:20R

6x50 pull (L3) w/:10R

[Continued on next page]

4x200 pull w/:30R;
  1 (L3)
  2 (L4)
  3 (L3)
  4 (L5)

4x50 freestyle; 25 (L5)/25 (L2) w/:10R

2x100 kick alternate; 25 (L4)/25 (L2) w/:20R

2x100 pull; 25 (L4)/75 (L2) w/:20R

8x25 freestyle; odds (L5), evens (L3) w/:10R

100 choice of stroke (L2)

TOTAL: 4800

L1: Recovery; L2: Aerobic; L3: High-End Aerobic to Low Anaerobic;
L4: Lactate or Anaerobic Threshold; L5: Sub-Maximum to Maximum Effort

21

300 freestyle (L2)
200 kick (L2)

200 pull (L2)

2x:

    4x25 alternate; fist drill/freestyle w/:15R

    75 pull (L4)

    2x50 6-3-6 drill w/:15R

    75 kick; 25 breast/25 flutter/ 25 back (L2)

100 kick (L3)
100 kick on back (L3)
100 6-3-6 drill
100 pull (L3)

[Continued on next page]

4x100 freestyle (L5) broken at the 50 for :05 w/:20R

50 freestyle (L2)

3x100 freestyle (L5) broken at the 75 for :05 w/:20R

50 freestyle (L2)

2x100 freestyle (L5) w/:20R

50 freestyle (L5)

100 freestyle (L5)

50 freestyle (L2)

3x300 w/1:00R;
   1 pull build
   2 freestyle (L4)
   3 pull build

100 freestyle (L4)

100 kick (L2)

100 freestyle (L4)

100 pull (L2)

4x150 freestyle descend the set
   w/:30R

100 choice of stroke (L2)

TOTAL: 5000

22

300 freestyle (L2)
200 kick (L2)

200 pull (L2)
10x50; 25 catch-up drill/25 freestyle w/:15R
8x25 6-3-6 drill w/:10R
4x25 fist drill w/:10R
4x25 stroke count w/:10R
4x25 finger tip drag drill w/:10R

4x50 kick (L3) w/:15R
100 6-3-6 drill
150 pull (L3)
100 kick (L4)
4x50 pull (L3) w/:15R

L1: Recovery; L2: Aerobic; L3: High-End Aerobic to Low Anaerobic;
L4: Lactate or Anaerobic Threshold; L5: Sub-Maximum to Maximum Effort

2x400 w/1:00R;

   1 freestyle (L4)

   2 pull breathe every 3rd (L3)

4x:

   100 freestyle fastest time w/:10R

   50 your choice freestyle or kick (L2)

   1:00R between each set

8x75 freestyle; 25 (L2)/25 (L4)/25 (L2) w/:15R

9x50; odds backstroke, evens freestyle (L2) w/:15R

100 choice of stroke (L2)

TOTAL: 5000

23

300 freestyle (L2)
200 kick (L2)

200 pull (L2)
8x25 catch-up drill w/:10R
3x50 freestyle build each w/:10R
150 pull build

200; 100 IM/100 freestyle (L3)
2x75 freestyle descend the set
     w/:20R
2x75; 25 butterfly/25 backstroke/
     25 breaststroke w/:15R

100 kick (L2)
2x100 kick (L4) w/:15R
50 choice (L2)

L1: Recovery; L2: Aerobic; L3: High-End Aerobic to Low Anaerobic;
L4: Lactate or Anaerobic Threshold; L5: Sub-Maximum to Maximum Effort

300 (L4)

50 pull (L2)

100 freestyle (L2)

4x50 freestyle (L5) w/:20R

200 pull (L3)

4x50 freestyle (L5) w/:20R

2x100 freestyle (L5) w/:15R

50 choice (L2)

300 pull (L3)

50 breaststroke (L2)

200 kick (L2)

3x50 kick (L3) w/:10R

50 freestyle (L2)

200 pull (L4)

3x50 freestyle (L5) w/:30R

50 kick (L2)

[Continued on next page]

200 freestyle (L4)
200 kick (L2)

100 choice of stroke (L2)

TOTAL: 5000

24

300 freestyle (L2)
200 kick (L2)

200 pull (L2)
3x50 catch-up drill w/:15R
3x50 6-3-6 drill w/:15R
3x50 kick (L2) w/:15R
150 pull (L2)

4x w/:10R:
 2x25 freestyle build each
 2x25 butterfly build each
 2x25 freestyle (L5)
 50 freestyle (L2)

3x w/:15R:
 100 freestyle (L4)

[Continued on next page]

4x25 pull (L3)

100 freestyle (L5)

4x25 pull (L3)

2x w/:15R:

2x100 freestyle; 25 (L4)/25 (L2)/ 25 (L5)/25 (L2)

2x25 kick (L3)

4x25 freestyle (L4)

300 pull locomotion

200 freestyle (L4)

200 freestyle (L5)

100 kick (L2)

200 choice of stroke (L2)

TOTAL: 5000

L1: Recovery; **L2**: Aerobic; **L3**: High-End Aerobic to Low Anaerobic;
L4: Lactate or Anaerobic Threshold; **L5**: Sub-Maximum to Maximum Effort

25

300 freestyle (L2)

200 kick (L2)

200 pull (L2)

2x50; 25 6-3-6 drill/25 catch-up drill w/:15R

3x50 kick (L3) w/:15R

3x50 pull (L3) w/:15R

3x50; 25 6-3-6 drill/25 finger tip drag drill w/:15R

150 freestyle (L3) w/:15R

200 pull (L3) w/:15R

1000 freestyle alternate; 100 (L4)/ 100 (L2)

200 kick (L2)

[Continued on next page]

2x100 freestyle alternate; 50 (L5)/ 50 (L2) w/:15

400 pull (L3)

50 freestyle (L3)

300 pull (L3)

50 freestyle (L3)

10x50 pull; odds (L3), evens (L4) w/:15

12x25 freestyle (L4) w/:15

4x75 freestyle; 50 (L4)/25 (L2) w/:15

100 choice of stroke (L2)

TOTAL: 5000

L1: Recovery; L2: Aerobic; L3: High-End Aerobic to Low Anaerobic;
L4: Lactate or Anaerobic Threshold; L5: Sub-Maximum to Maximum Effort

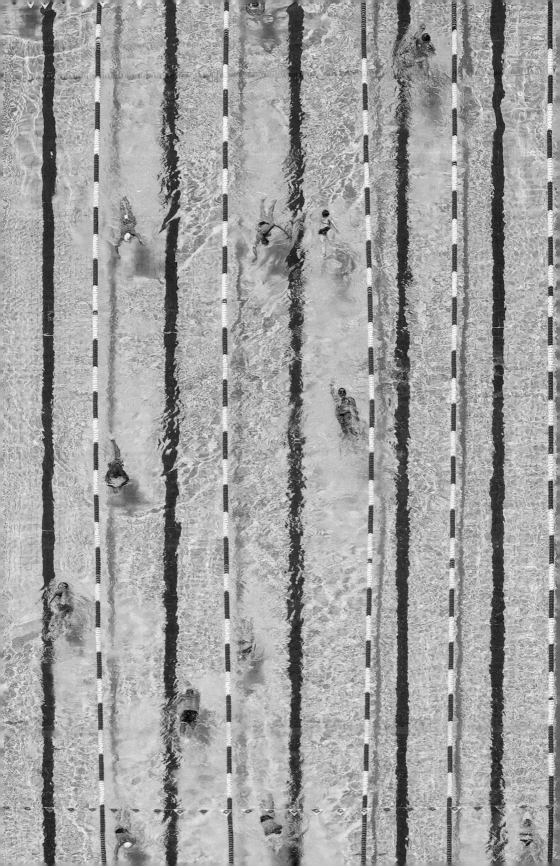

ABOUT THE AUTHOR

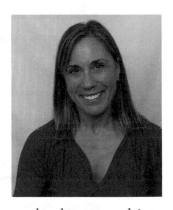

Terri Schneider is an ultra-endurance athlete, writer, speaker, coach and sport psychology consultant. She has authored *Dirty Inspirations: Lessons from the Trenches of Extreme Endurance Sports* and *Triathlon Revolution: Training, Technique and Inspiration,* co-authored *Triathlete's Guide to Mental Training,* and contributed to several other books. As a former 10-year professional triathlete focusing on the IRONMAN® distance, she then segued into adventure racing with the inception of the Eco Challenge in 1995, as well as ultrarunning and mountaineering. Terri earned a bachelors degree in exercise physiology as well as a masters degree in sport psychology with a research emphasis on risk taking and team dynamics. Her writing contributions, profile, and interviews have been featured in over 100 publications and websites around the world including Time, Psychology Today, Rolling Stone, Runner's World, Triathlete, Cosmopolitan, Glamour, Outside, Oxygen, USA Today, and The New York Times. While Santa Cruz, CA remains her home base, she spends time each year volunteering in Bhutan while continuing to explore and adventure around the globe, sharing her experiences through her speaking, writing and photography. For more info go to www.terrischneider.net.

ALSO IN THE SERIES

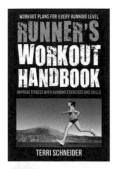

Runner's Workout Handbook
978-1-57826-697-5
E-Book: 978-1-57826-698-2

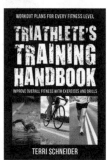

Triathlete's Training Handbook
978-1-57826-724-8
E-Book: 978-1-57826-725-5

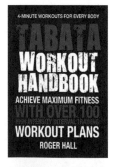

Tabata Workout Handbook
978-1-57826-561-9
E-Book: 978-1-57826-562-6

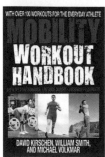

The Mobility Workout Handbook
978-1-57826-619-7
E-Book: 978-1-57826-620-3

getfitnow

GOT QUESTIONS?
NEED ANSWERS?
GO TO:
GETFITNOW.COM

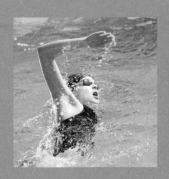 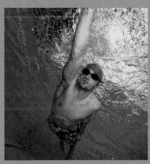 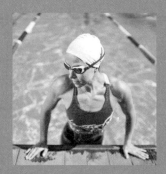

IT'S FITNESS 24/7

Videos, Workouts, Nutrition,
Recipes, Community Tips, and more!